TOO **BIG**:

A Guide for Coping when Pain Replaces Pleasure

Robert W. Birch, Ph.D.
ACS Certified Sexologist
(Retired Marital & Sex Therapist)

TOO BIG: A Guide for When Pain Replaces Pleasure

by

Robert W. Birch, Ph.D.
ACS Certified Sexologist

PEC Publishing®

http://www.oralcaress.com

ISBN-10 1449519792
ISBN-13   9781449519797

It was once said of a man
that his penis was so big
it required its own zip code.

TABLE OF CONTENTS

THEY COME IN ALL SIZES

Penises

We all know that penises, like noses, come in all sizes, shapes and the directions in which they point. Some erections point up, some point down, some left and some right – and, of course, there are a lot that point straight out. There are unique twists to some, bends and curves. Often the head is bigger than the circumference of the shaft, some times it is the same diameter and sometime the head is dwarfed by the shaft's thickness. Of all the various characteristics of the male penis, the one that gets the most attention is size!

Many men worry about their size and seem to worry a lot more than most women worry about it. Most women would agree that a man's ability to make mad passionate love has a lot more to do with his skill and sensuality than with the size of his erection. Still, men continue to worry and there are also women who help perpetuate the belief that bigger is *always* better.

One of the misunderstandings that contributes to the societal obsession with size is the belief that all women should reach orgasm during intercourse and penis size is the key. In reality, only about thirty-five percent of orgasmic women ever climax during intercourse, and typically only in positions in which they also are receiving clitoral stimulation. Penis size is not the critical factor. Knowledge is.

Realistically, however, there are the issues of fit. Penises come in all sizes but so do vaginas. Some penises fit better in some vaginas than they do in others. Yes, some women comment on penises that are too small or too thin, but in terms of complaints in the office of most sex therapists, the greatest number of size complaints focus on those that are just too big – too long, too fat or both.

Vaginas

Let's spend a little time considering the nature of what some have called the "love tunnel." When the vagina is relaxed, the vaginal walls collapse down to each other. The diameter of the non- aroused vagina barrel is less than one inch and its length will be around three to four inches. However, the size changes with arousal. With sexual excitement the diameter of the vagina expands, although not the same throughout the length of the vaginal tunnel.

The narrowest part will be around the opening of vagina, known as the *entroitus*. This vestibule is surrounded by muscles and is from one to two inches in length. Beyond this muscular opening the diameter becomes wider as it goes deeper. Usually the front part of vagina has a size of one and a half inches, but the back-end of the tunnel will balloon out to a diameter of about two and a half inches. This is in part due to the pulling up of the uterus and cervix, creating what has been called the "tenting effect." The length of the vaginal barrel also changes with arousal, extending itself from about three and a half inches to four or more inches. However, the size will be changed some after child birth because of the extreme expansion of the vagina. As with measurements of penis length and girth, the numbers for vaginal length and diameter vary as well.

Most women easily accommodate an average-size erection, usually defined as between five and a half and six and a half inches. However, an extremely thick penis of average length can be problematic. Some claim a woman with an average-size vagina can handle an erection nine inches long and two inches wide. This might, however, be depended on the woman's level of arousal, abundance of lubrication and position of intercourse, as well as her vaginal size. It has been estimated that 60 percent of women have a normal size vagina, but 10 percent are smaller and 30 percent are larger.

It is important to understand that the vagina is not an open tube. The walls, which have the potential to expand and elongate, gently touch one another even during arousal. When something is placed inside, they mold around the width and accommodate the length of a penis, tampon, finger(s), or sex toy. Unfortunately there are limits to the ability to expand, dependent not only on penis size, but the woman's degree of arousal, her level of relaxation and the extent of her anxiety.

Sometimes during intercourse, a penis does hit the cervix. This may be an indication that the woman is not excited enough. Remember, when a woman is more aroused, her vagina will elongate and her cervix will lift up and move out of the way. Other times, contact with the cervix can happen if a penis is larger than average or if the thrusting is too deep.

With a long penis it might feel like something internal is being bumped into to. The other dimension that can be problematic is diameter. Some erections are too fat for the woman and she experiences penetration as very painful. She will describe this as a painful stretching. One man said to me, "But they'll stretch enough for a baby to go through," and I asked him "But how many women have described delivery as physically pleasurable?" Sex should be fun, not labor.

Both men and women believe a tighter vagina will bring greater pleasure to both parties, its walls providing more pressure and friction. On the other hand, tightness can certainly contribute to the problem of incompatible sizes if the man is too large.

Painful Intercourse and Penis Size

When a woman experiences painful intercourse, the joy goes out of the act. She might then begin to avoid the experience and this could have a serious impact on her relationship. Still, however, companies continue to sell penis enlargement pills, patches, potions and pumps because men continue to want something bigger and are willing to waste money on these products. Despite the claims and testimonials, there are no proven ways to enlarge a penis! Still the "add inches" hype continues while a lot of women just want a man who knows how to make sensual love to her mind and to her body without inflicting pain.

Of course there are women who will say they want a one big, for as I have said, vaginas come in all sizes too. A large woman with a large vagina might easily handle something big, but it would not be easy for an average-sized woman with an average-sized vagina. Still, the image of the large penis draws attention, draws admiration by some and causes a lot of men to worrying themselves sick and spend a lot of money trying to gain something they will never achieve. And the question should be asked of these men, "What would you do with something that is too big for most women to handle?"

This is not a guide about running from the man you love or desire because he is well-hung. This is about how to enjoy sexual pleasures, albeit with some modifications and restrictions. A woman with a big partner already knows she will not enjoy the penetration if she is not fully relaxed and highly aroused. She also knows she cannot lie on her back, legs wide open and have her men pound hard and deep into her.

Sexual Pain (*Dyspareunia*)

Before talking about relaxation, maintaining arousal and alternate positions, let's talk more about sexual pain. The medical term for pain during intercourse is ***dyspareunia***, from Greek meaning '*Unhappily mated as bedfellows.*' There is hope, however, but let's first talk of discomfort. Pain with intercourse can occur at the opening into the vagina, within the walls of the vaginal canal, at its far end or any combination of locations. [Many use the term *vagina* to refer to all of a woman's genitals, but technically the *vagina* is only the tunnel and everything else is her *vulva*.] The pain within the vagina can be experienced as localized or generalized, as sharp or dull, and can be described as a stretching, burning, or stabbing sensation. The pain might be within the vagina itself or off to one side of the abdomen. There can also be pain within the vulva. Since physical discomfort is not always related to the size of a partner, the best understanding of sexual pain is always gained by detailed discussion with a gynecologist, follow by a thorough pelvic examination.

Recognizing the limitations of this impersonal guide, consider these general thoughts. A stretching sensation at the vaginal opening is often associated with the entry of a thick erection and/or the woman not being fully relaxed and/or highly aroused and lubricated. A burning sensation along the walls of the vagina is often caused by decreased lubrication as the result of incomplete arousal, or the estrogen depletion associated with menopause. Vagina walls tend to dry, thin and lose their elasticity with menopausal hormonal changes, especially if there has been a decrease in the woman's sexual activity.

A long erection is likely to be the cause of stretching at the far end of the vaginal canal and it is possibly accompanied with the feeling of having something in the abdomen bumped into. Pain off to one side or the other, especially if it is occasional and alternates sides each month, might simply be a sensitive ovary that is about to pop an egg. Again, sexual pain within the vulva or vagina or anywhere in the abdomen should always be discussed in detail with a physician.

The Sexual Response

Sex is not simple and sexual pain is complicated, so here's one more informational side-track to help put things into perspective. The full sexual response begins with feelings of *desire*. With stimulation (psychological and/or physical) there is then the building of *arousal*, and with effective physical stimulation everything ends gloriously with *orgasm*. So, a woman begins by feeling horny, gets turned on and with her excitement she lubricates, and eventually has at least one orgasm (generally with clitoral stimulation). Typically a woman must feel secure and relaxed to respond, and many women would add needing to feel emotionally close.

During the process of arousal, along with the appearance of lubrication, the muscles surrounding the opening into a woman's vagina begin to relax and the opening opens. The vaginal walls also open and the canal actually lengths by a half inch or more, but even at that it remains relatively short. Nature prepares the woman for intercourse.

Ideally the response sequence begins with desire, which is the motivator, the libido, the starter. This is the initial incentive to seek sexual stimulation and arousal. However, under the right circumstances it is often possible to skip the desire and jump-start arousal. If the starter is not working it does not automatically mean the motor will not run. In order to jump-start arousal the woman needs to be willing, relaxed, secure, and many would add loved. Of equal importance is a slow and patient approach with effective mental and physical stimulation. More will be said later about getting a jump-start when the starter is being sluggish (low or absent libido).

Negative Cycles

If there is sexual pain, the anticipation of that discomfort can dampen a woman's desire and interfere with her arousal. She is likely to begin avoiding or postponing sexual encounters, and as a result her partner might experience a more pressing desire to penetrate when finally given the opportunity. If foreplay is rushed or is ineffective, the woman will not become well lubricated, especially if she is postmenopausal. If she is not relaxed and sufficiently wet, this will add to the pain she experiences.

A cycle might begin: She feels pain and then begins to anticipate and to fear that uncomfortable predictable experience. As a result of the anxiety, she remains physically tense, slow to arousal and relatively dry. If tight, not sufficiently aroused and well lubricated, she is likely to experiences more pain, and her fears of greater future discomfort increases her apprehension and reinforces her avoidance.

Unfortunately, many women say their partner only will touch them when he thinks it will lead to intercourse and orgasm. Sexual avoidance is not uncommon when there is pain, and so a lot of women with partners, only come to bat when they think they can score a home run, feel they must avoid all touch, lest the man become aroused and press for intercourse.

Now we see the cycle a man can get into: He wants sex, approaches but feels rejected. He still wants sex, and this time he's advances are accepted. He rushes to intercourse, she feels pain and rejects his next offer. His pressure on the woman increases and her avoidance multiplies in response. This is perceived by the man as rejection, he becomes angry, she loses interest in being sexual with an angry man and the risk of a very destructive couple's cycle develops, with neither partner being able to identify the steps.

A relationship cycle can begin anywhere. It might begin with the woman fearing pain and rejecting the man's sexual advances. The man might then react with anger and he in turn neglects the woman emotionally. In response to his anger and neglect, the woman's interest in being sexual with him decreases and she is set up to reject him when he again expresses an interest in sex.

With a cycle, however, the chain of events could have started with the man being angry about something else and cutting off his affection. In response the woman's desire for him weakens and she then rejects his sexual advances. This only makes him more angry and neglectful and she is even less inclined to make love.

When a man only touches a woman when he wants sex and once started he presses for intercourse, if pain results, the fear of discomfort enters the cycle, impacting the woman both emotionally and physically. The same is true if the man is clumsy, awkward or lacks sensuality in his approach. If he fails to arouse the woman fully and she becomes apprehensive, there is an increase in the risk that intercourse will be painful.

Out of fear the woman is likely to begin to avoid another such encounter. The man will react and his reaction will impact the relationship.

Fear is reduced if the anxiety-arousing situation is totally avoided. Cycles are hard to break, especially when avoidance has become a way to decrease anxiety.

When there is a burning sensation within the vagina due to lack of lubrication, anxiety might again be the culprit. If a woman is not mentally and physically relaxed, her arousal will be diminished, lost or completely blocked. Without arousal there is no lubrication and without sufficient lubrication intercourse can be painful. When the fear of pain kicks in, cycles begin.

Recap on Sexual Pain

Sex is not supposed to hurt, but for many women it does. There are many medical reasons for painful intercourse (clinically called dyspareunia), and a physician should always be consulted. Pain might occur around the lips and clitoris, right around the vaginal opening or deep within the vagina or abdomen. The pain might be experienced as a burning sensation, a sharp pain, a stretching experience or a dull ache. It might occur during entry (entry dyspareunia) or deep (bumper dyspareunia).

Women should be willing to talk with their medical doctors in detail, describing the location of the pain, the nature of the pain, and the activities that trigger the discomfort. Most gynecologists have heard it all and will know what to look for during the pelvic exam.

There are some women who, even though aroused, do not lubricate well. This might be due to age or medications that are being taken, or just something about the woman's biology. If this dryness is all it is, the problem is likely to be solved with the use of a good, safe, water-soluble lubricant such as Astroglide® or Slippery Stuff®. There are many other good sexual lubricants on the market.

There are a number of medical conditions that will cause sharp localized pain within the genital lips or around the vaginal opening, or a burning sensation along the vaginal walls. Persistent deep pain, or pain that seems related to a woman's monthly cycle, should be discussed with a physician. This type of pain and problems with lubrication might require medical attention.

To help clarify in her own mind the information about her discomfort that would aid in her diagnosis and treatment, before consulting her doctor a woman should think about describing her pain. Is it chronic (long term) or acute (of recent onset)? Does it occur only during intercourse, also during sex play or at times totally unrelated to sexual activity? Where is it felt? Is it external, just at the very opening, within the muscular entroitus, inside the vaginal barrel, at the far end or some combination of locations? Is something being bumped into? If it is a deep pain, is it midline or off to the right or left, and is the location consistent?

What kind of pain or discomfort is it? Do you feel stretched? Is it a burning sensation, a sharp localized pain or a dull ache. If there have recently been several partners, has the discomfort occurred with each, and if not, is there some characteristic of the man or men who have inflicted pain. Is it length, girth, perhaps a bend or angle to their erection or a combination. The woman will also need to tell of her level of arousal and of the quantity and quality of her lubrication. If a woman needs to talk about her sexual pain to a sex therapist or to her gynecologist, she should not keep any secrets.

Vaginismus

Vaginismus is one cause of sexual pain, but can also be the result of it. Let's identify a negative cycles triggered by an over-sized penis and the incompatibility of fit with the woman. When there is discomfort, there is a risk of a possible *psychosomatic* consequence. Pain on penetration can generate an emotional fear of intercourse, as we have stated, but it can also trigger a reflexive and unconscious constriction of the muscles around the opening of the vagina. This involuntary constriction can become chronic and is referred to as *vaginismus*.

If there is a history of pain that stirs a woman's fear of penetration, with a tighter vaginal opening that pain will be exacerbated. The greater the pain, the greater the fear and the more likely the avoidance. The unconscious tightening has been likened to the eyes blinking reflex, a built in defense reaction. Simply avoiding intercourse does not resolve the vaginismus.

With severe cases of vaginismus, penetration with a small penis, a finger or even a tampon might become impossible. In such persistent and extreme cases the therapeutic intervention of a qualified sex therapist is generally required. Information on understanding sex therapy is included in this book's Appendix.

Relaxation and Non-Demand Pleasuring

The questions becomes, how can a couple begin to break destructive cycles that are preventing them from dealing directly and creatively with the pain? Penis size cannot be changed, but the anxiety it causes can be reduced and a woman can learn to relax and allow her body to respond. If the pain of intercourse has resulted in vaginismus or intense anxiety, and has dampened desire and weakened arousal, the first step is obvious. Stop the painful act. Stop having intercourse! Don't panic, however, for this moratorium is temporary. It's an investment in a future of pain-free sexual play.

The prohibition against intercourse, included in the sex therapist's first "homework" assignment, is not a "do-not-touch" mandate. In fact, the couple should plan to touch at least twice a week. By planning ahead, the sessions are not rushed, last-minute, late-at-night events as sexual encounters often are. Time should be built in for showering or bathing so that each starts out feeling clean and relaxed. The couple should then take turns sensually massaging each other, starting on backs and, if agreed upon, then fronts. However, breasts and genitals should be off limits. The initial goal is not to arouse, and even if arousal occurs, the prohibitions should remain in place. The goal is not intercourse or orgasms. The goal is relaxation!

The woman's fear and anxiety that had developed were caused by her anticipation of genital pain. With penetration off limits, there are no pressures, no demands and no threat of physical discomfort. There is no worry about having to become aroused or having to deal with the size issue, and there is time to experience a pleasurable full-body nonsexual massage. Add to the sensual ambience of the experience by lighting aromatic candles and playing soft background music. Use a scented massage oil, warmed first in a pan of warm water. Be gentle – this should be a sensual massage, not a therapeutic one.

The receiver is to lie quietly and say nothing as long as the touch is pleasurable and relaxing. The giver is urged to experience the temperatures and textures of the partner's body, focus on the sensations of touch, hearing, smelling and sight. The giver should experience the sensual process of giving and not focus on turning on the receiver. In sex therapy this homework is known as *Sensate Focus*, and **Step One** was described above.

After a couple of weeks of trading back and forth who gets to receive first, but only if the desired comfort and relaxation has occurred, move on to **Step Two**. In this second step, breasts and genitals remain off limits. Relaxation when receiving and pleasure when giving remain, but another goal is added – learning to give feedback. The receiver now has the responsibility to share information on how he or she likes to be touched. It is important, however, that the feedback remain positive, as in, "I like being touched gently on that spot. Yes, that feels much better," as opposed to the negative "You're touching me wrong there!" Moans are also a way to signal pleasure. The receiver can also give nonverbal feedback by placing a hand on the giver's hand and gently moving it to an area that feels better.

This can also be a time for the giver to express his or her pleasure in giving. Talk of the textures experienced, the contours enjoyed and the variations in temperature found.

After a couple of weeks, if relaxation continues and feedback has been found helpful, move onto **Step Three**. Breasts now come on limits, but genitals and intercourse remain off. With the moratoriums in place, the caressing of the breasts should be more for the sensual pleasure of giver and receiver, rather than a step in the progress ending with penetration. Include the breasts as a part of the total body, without giving them a lot of extra attention. Verbal feedback by the woman is important in this step. If erotic feelings occur, fine. If not, fine. Learn to touch and be touched in erogenous areas without feeling the need for building excitement or coital completion. Find pleasure in giving and receiving sensual caress.

As the goal is the woman's relaxation, she must remaintain in control. If at any point her anxiety begins to build, she should ask her partner to back up. If she is able to relax again, she can then ask him to continue. However, if she remains anxious, the session should end. It is okay to say, "Let's stop for now." This is a valuable lesson. Whenever anxiety occurs, back off and reestablish the relaxation. Do not attempt to press through anxiety, as that usually only adds more pressure.

After two weeks (at least four sessions), with the woman's permission move to **Step Four.** By now many couples will remark, "We've had a lot less sex, but we've sure done a lot more touching." In this fourth step breasts and genitals (his and hers) are on limits, but intercourse remains off limits. The goals remains relaxation and the effective exchange of information. In this step you will better appreciate the benefits of verbal feedback, for it is more important to tell how you like your genitals caressed than to tell how to stroke your feet.

It is important to do the full-body massage before approaching genital areas, and the woman's vulva should not be touched without her permission. If she is feeling any anxiety, the caress of her genitals should be postponed. She needs also to closely monitor her feelings about caressing her partner's penis. In any case, the goal is not orgasm. The touch could be light and experimental.

The giver should concentrate on the textures of the partner's genitals and listen carefully to the feedback. If the receiver is silent, the giver can ask something like, "Do you like it here better than here?" "How do you like this spot touched?" The receiver then gives non-critical feedback. "That feels good and lighter would feel even better."

The massage oil should not be used on the woman's vulva, as we don't know what might be growing in the oil. Instead, switch to a safe, water soluble lubricant such as *Astroglide*. With a sexual lubricant, have the bottle warming in a pan of warm water. The massage oil can, however, be used on the man's penis and should prove pleasurable for both giver and receiver. Remember, the goal is to learn and not to trigger an orgasm.

In this step the woman's arousal might occur if she is relaxed and if the clitoral caress is gentle and on target. Without pressure to perform and with effective feedback, she is likely to turn on and begin to lubricate. At this point the stimulation of her vulva and clitoris, however, should not lead to any vaginal penetration.

It will be helpful to understand that there are two types of sexual arousal: *Psychogenic* and *Reflexogenic*. Psychogenic arousal is getting turned on with fantasy, memories, seeing a desired partner, nonsexual touch or just a hormonal surge. The genesis (beginning) is primarily in the psyche or mind. Reflexogenic arousal, on the other hand, begins as a physical response to direct stimulation of erogenous areas of the body. It is a biological reflex, and this type of excitement has also been called *biogenic* arousal.

Very often a woman will not begin to respond until there is non-demand pleasurable touch on and around her clitoris, and a warm slippery lubricant sure helps. This is the "jump-start" mechanism that can begin from scratch, even without prior desire. However, it requires comfort, relaxation, a slow approach and effective stimulation. If the starter is not working, it is still possible to get the motor running with the loving boost from a jump start..

Recapping so far: Hopefully at this point in the Sensate Focus process, the couple has learned the value of planning and setting aside time, during which the touching is not foreplay, but for play. In the process, the value of open communication will hopefully be understood and appreciated. With effective communication, each should be learning how best to touch the partner and finding pleasure in giving pleasure. Most important for the woman is not feeling vulnerable being nude, gaining comfort with being touched without fear of pain and learning to be in control. At this point, however, there has been no penetration.

Divide this step of genital touching into two parts, and for the first week touch genitals to relax, communicate and learn. If this goes well for two sessions, and if the woman feels aroused, lubricated and ready, for the next two sessions she can ask for finger penetration. Remember, this is only after there has been full body massage and effective caress of her vulva and clitoris. The penetration should be slow and easy with one finger. There can be some gentle thrusting as long as there is no pain. Circular movement should indicate something of the relaxation of the muscles surrounding the vaginal opening. With permission, two fingers can be inserted. If there is discomfort or if anxiety begins to build, the woman must identify this verbally to her partner. The giver should back up, withdrawing his fingers and returning to a gentle clitoral caress.

However, if there is comfort and if the woman is aroused and willing, now would be a good time to learn if she is responsive to *G Spot* stimulation. Some women are, but not all, and the majority of those who are will report they still have a preference for clitoral attention. But, this is an area of curiosity and another opportunity to playfully explore and exchange information.

To reach the G Spot insert two fingers (with palm up) and curl then up behind the woman's pubic bone. Then to stroke the area, which will feel spongy, finger tips are moved as though signaling someone to "come here."

To the woman this might feel pleasurable, it might feel annoying, or she might feel nothing at all. Very few women would ever orgasm with G Spot stimulation alone. Return to clitoral stimulation and talk about the different sensations. Find pleasure in trying new things and exchanging information about the experience.

In this second part of this step, <u>orgasms are allowed, but not required</u>! Keep the emphasis on relaxation and non-demand pleasuring. Do not turn this phase into work – let happen what will happen and regardless of where it ends up, if there has been pleasure and relaxation consider it a success. This portrays an approach to physical intimacy that is good for a lifetime. It is a *failsafe philosophy* that says there is not failure if your goals remain pleasure and relaxation. It is the way to literally stay in touch for a lifetime.

Recapping, the Senate Focus steps have hopefully removed the anxiety over penetration by removing that possibility. In the process of the non-demand pleasuring, information has then been exchanged, sensual and sexual pleasure has been experienced, and the jump-start approach to reflexogenic arousal has been explored. Hopefully the value of setting aside time for non-demand play is beginning to make sense. A metaphor told by sex therapists to illustrate this principle is presented in the Appendix.

Failsafe Sexuality

To better understand the concept of failsafe sexuality, consider all the sensual options with a non-goal directed approach. One can begin with any sensual or sexual activity, but with this philosophy there is no end goal that must be reached. There is no set path that must be followed and no pressure to finish with orgasms. While intercourse might be included in your menu, it need not always be the goal or the only activity. There are many ways to "make love," and variety can add to the excitement. If intercourse is not automatically the goal each playtime, there is no sense of failure if it does not occur.

One might choose to begin with snuggling or sharing some sexual fantasy and a bit of gentle play of each other's genitals might be added. That could be it. On another occasion during a sensual massage, a couple might take time to visually explore each other's body and end up with an exchange of oral sex, talking along the way of sights, aromas and tastes.

Reading erotica or watching an erotic DVD might lead to some self-stimulation, either alone or together. With the failsafe approach, whatever happens is a success, for without specific goals there can be no failure.

There are many sensual and sexual options available to a creative couple. In coping with an incompatibility in size, both man and woman must maintain effective communication as they explore new ways of relating sexually. Trust me, the purpose of this guide is not to ban intercourse from the list of options. The purpose is to work toward pain-free and mutually pleasurable intimacy, and a fail-safe philosophy that is good for a lifetime!

The Woman Alone

There is an important task most women should undertake if their partner's erection is thick and has caused pain on penetration. The first step is for the woman to practice relaxing her entire body. Relaxation or music CDs might help. A woman needs then to focus in and become fully aware of those muscles surrounding her vaginal opening.

Once she is certain she has relaxed her pelvic floor muscles, that band of muscles that stretches between her legs, she is ready for the next task. These muscles around the entroitus are called the "pubococcygeal muscles" because the stretch from the pubic bone in front, back to the coccyx bone in back (the tail bone). They have been called the PC muscles for short. One female author referred to them as the "love muscle."

Within this band of muscles are those surrounding the vaginal opening and, it is interesting to note, these are the muscles that contract during orgasm. The woman's next task, after locating these muscles in her mind and relaxing them, is to voluntarily squeeze her vaginal opening. Once she has intentionally tightened these muscles she will discover that they automatically begin to relax. As they do, she should then concentrate on achieving complete relaxation. After a minute or two she should again squeeze these muscles tight and repeat the sequence several times a day.

This process is know as the Kegel Exercise, named after Dr. Arnold Kegel who was the first to identify them and write of their significance in improving the bladder control of older women.

It has been recommended that women associate this exercise (called *Kegeling*) with a daily activity, perhaps while watching the morning news, talking on the phone or stopping at the stop lights on the way to work. The idea, of course, is to have reminders to squeeze and relax these important PC muscles.

Some women have trouble mentally finding this muscular band. The easiest way to identify them is to consciously stop the flow during urination. The muscles used to stop the stream of urine are the PC muscles. So, why is it that a woman should learn to contract and relax her pelvic floor if she is not having bladder problems? These are the muscles that will <u>automatically</u> tighten in response to a woman's fear of painful penetration. It helps to know where they are, for it is helpful learning to relax a muscle if you can first voluntarily contract it. A bonus is a woman's orgasms might begin feeling more intense. You will find a recap of this information plus more on the Kegel exercises in this book's Appendix.

Taking Ownership

It is essential for all women to own their sexuality. That means they need to give up any notion that men are the experts and only a man can turn them on and bring them to orgasm. Women should be comfortable with masturbation, especially if they have been avoiding partner sex and have had difficulty relaxing with their man.

During self-stimulation a woman has the opportunity to learn about her sexual anatomy and her sexual response without feeling watched or evaluated. To tell a man what feels good requires the woman to first find out on her own. So, during the early non-sexual stages of the Sensate Focus process, or if the partner is away or there is no partner, a woman can be arousing and satisfying herself. It is also a time when she can learn about jump-starting her own arousal motor, and is also an opportunity to fantasize about pleasurable intercourse. Imagine the joy or recall making love with a previous better-fitting partner.

A woman's sexual arousal is important for the next steps in her homework. She should buy a number of dildos of a variety of sizes, from the smallest she can find to one that is close to the size of her partner. During masturbation, when fully relaxed, aroused and well lubricated, she should insert the smallest, being fully aware of the initial penetration. To best experience this, she should hold the tip of the dildo against the opening into her vagina, but should then squeeze tight and relax three times. As she relaxes the third time she can press a bit and at some point in her relaxation the smallest dildo should slide in. Once in, she should leave it in place and squeeze her muscles around it – then relax. If that goes well she can then move up to the next size.

With each increase in size, the procedure should be the same. First relax, then tighten. Place the tip at the opening, apply a bit of pressure and relax. Squeeze and relax three times before sliding in the dildo. The woman's goal is to become comfortable with the feeling of containment and to reassure herself that penetration is not necessarily painful.

At some point the size of the dildo should be as close as possible, in length and girth, to the partner's penis. I would recommend dildos that are softer than the hard plastic dildos or vibrators made for insertion. A flexible well-lubricated dildo is more "user friendly." Warming it first in warm water might add to the pleasure.

Now would be a time for a woman to experiment with a vibrator for <u>clitoral</u> stimulation. Combining vibrator stimulation with dildo vaginal containment might be a new and exiting experience for some. Mention will be made later about using a vibrator during pain-free positions of intercourse. This is helpful for women who can orgasm with vibrator stimulation of the clitoris, but not from intercourse alone, as is true for the majority of women.

In her alone time, a woman has the opportunity to explore her world of fantasy and build a repertoire of hot favorites. Sexual fantasies can serve three purposes: They can help ignite the flames of arousal, maintain the heat of arousal and facilitate the explosion of an orgasm. Sexual fantasies are also a good way to block anxiety, so it is worth exploring this erotic mental resource. Some women find fantasy material in erotic novels, while other prefer the tamer romantic genre. More on the topic of sexual fantasy will be found in the Appendix of this book.

Outercourse

Let's first look at coping with the thick penis. A step needs to be added and it involves what is known as *outercourse*. It is so named because the genital contact is <u>outside</u> the vagina.

For outercourse it is best if the man lies on his back. When he does so the sensitive softer underside of his erection is up. After applying a healthy layer of artificial lubrication to her partner's penis the woman straddles him. She then lowers herself, wiggling a bit if necessary to get him <u>between</u> the *labia* (lips) of her vulva.

She can sit a while and allow her partner to visually enjoy her body. He would also have the opportunity to caress her breasts. She should then lean forward a bit so that her clitoris makes better contact with his erection. The man remains passive while the woman slides back and forth. Perhaps for the first time his entire penis is being stimulated, albeit just on one side. This can provide very pleasurable feelings for both the man and the woman, and with a little practice both might orgasm in the process.

Once the woman is comfortable with her top position it is time to try another position of outercourse that works well with a thick penis. The woman is on her back with her legs up high. Her vulva is turned upward. The man can help by holding her legs up with his hands or even placing them on his shoulders. He then lays his erection between her well lubricated vulvar lips and slides. No penetration is made, but the man now feels in control, experiences the internal feedback of his pelvic thrusting and is often able to ejaculate in this position. The woman can maneuver just enough to get her clitoris involved.

One advantage to having outercourse as a step before intercourse is that it is another way a woman can learn to relax with her partner when he has more control. Most important is the opportunity for her to relax with their genitals in close proximity and not need to worry about penetration.

Pain-Free Intercourse with a Thick Penis

Despite everything said about de-emphasizing intercourse as the ultimate goal of sex play, most couples want to keep it high on their list of sexual options. If a couple has taken the Sensate Focus steps and the woman is relaxed and confident, and the man is more sensual and patient, and if the woman has practiced with dildos of increasing diameter and length, they are ready to more on.

That was a lot of ifs, but dealing with a thick penis is more of a problem than coping with a long one. If the problem is length, positions can be adjusted. When the problem is circumference, it is the woman who must adjust, and there are physical limits dependent on their relative sizes. A woman who complained of painful intercourse sat in my office holding a can of Coke. When I asked her how big the shaft of her partner's erection was she lifted the can. Her fingers did not completely circle the can. "He's not too long," she said, lifting the can higher, "but he's this thick."

When the partner's penis is thick, the best initial position for entry is the female superior (or woman on top) position. With the man lying passive on his back, the woman straddles him and he props up his erection. She then lowers her body to where the tip of the penis is just at the opening into her vagina. She then squeezes tight, holds it and relaxes. She should do this tightening and relaxing three times and the third time as she relaxes, she should take a deep breath and slowly press down onto the erection to the point where she feels discomfort. She is in control and no attempt for full penetration should be made, for this is a project that will take time.

Another position to experiment with is the standard "missionary position." The woman's legs are spread wide. There should be a lot of genitally focused foreplay with the woman in this position and she needs to be keeping track of her arousal, her anxiety level and her relaxation. If she stays in control she will feel more secure and not worry about a sneak attack. When she feels ready, and only then, she should squeeze her vaginal muscles tight and invite her partner to gently press the tip of his erection against her opening. Remember, it is often easier to relax muscles if one first focuses on them, and tensing these muscles serves this purpose. The muscles around the vaginal opening automatically being to relax when squeezed and held. This helps with the further relaxation of the PC muscles.

As these pelvic floor muscles being to relax, the woman should take a deep breath and relax as completely as possible. Once more, the process of tightening and relaxing should be repeated three times.

The man must then follow her directions. Once she feels relaxed, she can then invite penetration. "Gently," might be the agreed upon signal, or perhaps simply "Now." His entry should be slow and at the first sign of anxiety or pain or involuntary contraction she has two options. She can say "Stop" and attempt to relax with whatever degree of penetration there is, or she can say "Out," and he must withdraw immediately. They should agree in advance on the short *safe words* she will use so that her statement is immediately understood.

Perhaps the woman will be in the mood to try again if the first attempt is interrupted. If so, the man needs to back up and caress his partner in nonsexual areas. If she can begin to relax again, she can invite breast stimulation, and if still relaxed she can instruct him to caress her vulva and clitoris. When fully relaxed and well lubricated, she can again invite penetration, following the same squeeze and relax procedure, and with lots of verbal feedback. It will not help if the woman grits her teeth and passively allows herself to experience pain.

If the woman is not in the mood to attempt another penetration during that encounter, the couple should continue to play and, if agreed upon, help each other reach orgasm with outercourse, manual stimulation or oral sex. If the woman is comfortable with the insertion of two fingers, G Spot stimulation during *cunnilingus* can be very effective in triggering her climax. This combined stimulation is accomplished with the man between her legs, orally focusing on her clitoris. Two fingers are inserted palm down, but once the fingers are in, the man's hand is turned so his chin is resting in his palm. Curled fingertips reach the G Spot, located up behind her pubic bone.

When all of the steps are followed patiently and successfully, and penile penetration becomes pain-free, the man should avoid vigorous thrusting during the first dozen or more encounters. Then his pace and depth of thrusting can be negotiated. Women should always feel free to call off or modify the sexual encounter. Ultimately, however, it is the man's responsibility to protect his partner from physical pain, at times at the expense of being unable to ejaculate during intercourse.

Pain-Free Intercourse with a Long Penis

While nine or more inches might sound hot, most vaginas will not stretch comfortably to completely contain something of this length. With this size, uncontrolled hard thrusting in any position is likely to produce more pain than pleasure. Still, if the problem is length and not girth, position adjustments are possible to protect and pleasure the woman, and that is what will keep her coming back for more.

Following through the Sensate Focus process will help reduce a woman's anxiety and facilitate improved verbal and nonverbal communication. It will also introduce the concept of failsafe sensual and sexual intimacy. While intercourse is off limits, the woman can practice with dildos of various length, discovering on her own the depth to which she can be comfortably penetrated.

As the focus on non-demand pleasuring progresses, the couple should take advantage of some outercourse during their foreplay. This allows the woman to enjoy the full length of her partner's erection without having to worry about it causing her deep pain. Outercourse also provides the man with the sensations of the warm, wet, slippery vulva of his partner sliding along his entire shaft during this genital-to-genital caress. It is an opportunity for both partners to enjoy sexual intimacy without worrying about deep thrusting and bumper dyspareunia.

But, once intercourse is on limits, there are ways to achieve containment without pain. In the missionary position, once shallow vaginal penetration is made the woman can close her legs under her partner as he works his legs to the outside of her thighs. With her legs closed, it is usually unlikely that she will experience painful deep penetration, as not all of her partner's erection can enter. If this offers enough protection for the woman, he can safely thrust. If he slides higher on her body than he would if lying between her spread legs, he can angle the upper portion of his shaft down over her clitoris. This will add to her pleasure and, since most women need clitoral stimulation in order to orgasm, it will increase the likelihood she will climax with him inside.

In this modified missionary position, if the woman is well lubricate, either naturally or with additional artificial lubrication, with her legs closed and with him sliding over her clitoris, between her vulvar lips and into her vagina, he is likely to get the feeling of being completely encompassed. It could well be that he would find it difficult to distinguish what portion of his erection is actually outside his partner's body.

Some women wish to keep their legs open, but can usually spot an approaching missile that might hit bottom. In a new relationship she will have to decide quickly if it will be a comfortable fit. Since the missionary position is usually the first one couples try, a lot of women have figured out how to reach down and have long penises slide through their hand on the way into their vagina. Again, with lots of lubrication the man will likely feel totally involved, and the woman might enjoy, in addition to pain-free intercourse, the feeling of a firm penis sliding through her palm. Being experimental is important, but the goals should always be to play safe and have fun.

Any position that avoids full penetration will work, although clitoral stimulation might be limited. If the man is on his back and the woman squats over him, <u>facing his feet</u>, she can slide down to a depth that is comfortable to her. Then if she leans back, a portion of her partner's shaft will be denied entry. If his thrusting feels too deep, she can move back on his body. This would be a good position for the man to manually caress the woman's clitoris. If she were to lie back and off to one side, keeping him inside while freeing up her arms, she could reach down and stimulate herself or hold her favorite vibrator on her readily accessible clitoris.

Another safe position is the spoon position as long as it is a tight spoon, her back to his chest. If he was lying at a right angle to her body, his penetration would be deeper, so couples should experiment to determine which spooning arrangement works best for pain-free thrusting.

From the couple lying on their sides, if the woman were to roll over on her stomach, keeping her legs together, he could follow her over and her buttocks and thighs would hold him safely at bay. This is much safer than the doggie position with both on their knees.

Donuts

There is also a more mechanical approach, when a penis is too long. Complete penetration can be avoided through the use of soft "donuts," usually about an inch thick. One or more of these can be slid down to the base of the erection and, being soft, hard thrusting will not hurt either the man or the woman.

When length is the cause of the woman's discomfort, new positions should be explored and old ones modified. However, there are a number of positions that probably will not work without the use of these donuts! Sitting on the man's lap, face to face, without donuts will probably be risky if he is the owner of a long penis. Also, the rear- entry "doggie style" position is not on the menu for couples with a size discrepancy without the use of extreme care and the use of the donuts.

Three in Bed

A woman might want to experiment with taking both her partner and her vibrator to bed. As mentioned earlier, the majority of women will not orgasm with just vaginal stimulation, regardless of the size of her partner's equipment. Typically, direct clitoral stimulation is more effective than stimulation within the vagina. The female superior position, facing the man's feet, was mentioned as one position in which a vibrator can be use during intercourse. With the use of donuts, a woman can reach back under her body and hold a long-handled vibrator on her clitoris in the doggie position.

Another position to experiment with is the scissors position. The woman lies on her back and lifts her right leg. The man, lying at right angles to her body, slides under that leg and slides his legs around her left leg. Penetration can be made and it is easy to control the depth. In addition, it is not a position that allows the man to thrust rapidly. Many men enjoy being able to see their partner's upper body and women find it easy to reach down and stimulate their clitoris either with fingers or with their favorite toy.

Summary

If men get beyond thinking that making love is only about intercourse, and women are able to open up and explore new alternatives and positions, sex can move from pain to pleasure. Opening minds is more important than opening legs, and in lovemaking all of the senses should be involved. When time is made for play, there is time to experiences all the temperatures and textures of each others bodies. There is time to look, explore and appreciate the visual aspects of a lover's public and private areas. The aroma and tastes of a partner need be a part of the sensual experience, and sounds of pleasure should fill the room. Good sex is wet, good sex is noisy and good sex does not require deep penetration and marathon thrusting if the result is pain.

Appendix

THE KEGEL EXERCISES

A Little History

A band of muscles stretch between the legs of both men and women, stretching from the pubic bone in front to the coccyx (tail) bone in back. Playfully, we could say that with out these muscles, all of our internal organs would fall out! Along their way, this sling of muscles includes the sphincter of the bladder, the sphincter of the anus, and, in a woman, the sphincter surround the opening of her vagina. This important band of muscles are clinically known as the pubococcygeus (pronounced pew-bo-kak-se-gee'-us) muscles, but this group of muscles is more commonly called the "PC muscle." To talk as though there is just one muscle is an over-simplification, for there are actually a number of muscle groups that collectively make up this pelvic floor sling. We'll use the plural and call them the PC muscles.

Many younger women have been introduced to their PC muscles during a pregnancy or during a postpartum exam when they were advised to exercise these muscles in order to restore muscle tone following childbirth. Many older women have been introduced to their PC muscles because these are the muscles that are exercised to correct the condition known as urinary incontinence (the involuntary loss of urine when coughing, sneezing, etc.). In fact, the exercise of these PC muscles as a medical treatment for urinary incontinence was first proposed in1948 by the California gynecologist Dr. Arnold Kegel, for whom the exercises have been named.

In 1952, Dr. Kegel published a report in which he claimed that the women doing his exercises were becoming more easily, more frequently and more intensely orgasmic! As these are the muscles that contract rhythmically during orgasm in both males and females, it is not surprising, therefore, that sex therapists have emphasized the importance of these pelvic floor muscles that surround the vaginal opening and play a major role in the orgasmic response.

Thirty years after Dr. Kegel's article, sex therapist Bryce Britton wrote a book titled "THE LOVE MUSCLE," calling her publication "Every Woman's Guide to Intensifying Sexual Pleasure." Many people still refer to the PC muscles as the love muscle. Now, over 50 years after Dr. Kegel published his discovery, and after several decades of "prescribing" the Kegel exercises as a component in teaching women to become orgasmic (or more easily orgasmic), what can we say about "Kegeling" the love muscle? We can say that doing the exercises will tone up the sphincter of the bladder and might tighten the muscles around the opening of the vagina. We can also assume that any well-toned muscle will contract more powerfully than would a flabby muscle, and hence the likelihood of stronger orgasms with stronger PC muscles. We can report with confidence that some women squeeze their PC muscles, forcing blood down into their genital tissue, and in so doing can turn themselves on. A very small minority of women might even be able to bring themselves to orgasm exclusively with voluntary pelvic floor contractions. Finally, it is safe to say that a woman can add novelty to a sexual encounter by voluntarily squeezing her well-toned vaginal sphincter around her partner's penis, and this might be fun for both giver and receiver.

What can most confidently be said about the entire "PC muscle controversy" is that in doing Dr. Kegel's exercises, a woman will achieve closer contact with her pelvis, is more likely to take ownership of her internal and external genitalia, will strengthen the muscles that contract during orgasm, and is probably making an investment in her lifelong urinary control! Is it a major component in a woman becoming orgasmic? Probably not, but it is certainly something non-orgasmic women should include in their quest for the "Big O." It is a part of the learning package.

Doing the Kegel Exercise

In getting started with the Kegel exercise of the PC muscles, the first task for many women is to locate them. The best advice for finding the muscles is to do so while urinating. Sitting on the toilet with legs slightly spread, try to interrupt the stream of urine without bringing your legs together. Stop and start the flow a number of times, trying to sense those muscles that are involved. Once you can control the flow of your urine and can also find and squeeze them when not on the toilet, you have identified this band of important pelvic floor muscles.

Remember, these muscles are not located in your abdomen, nor are they in your thighs! Try to isolate the muscles so you can tighten them without flexing your "abs" and without putting tension in your legs. It might take time to fine-tune your ability to find, isolate and contract the muscles, so do not become discouraged if you have difficulty at first.

Once you know you have found your PC muscles, you will find that you can flex them ("Kegeling") most any time you choose and without being noticed by others who might be around you. Doing a series of Kegel exercises each day in the course of typical activities is most helpful. For women who drive or ride to and from work each day, a practical plan is to do a series of contractions at each red light encountered, or at each gas station passed, or in response to some other reminder. While watching TV, squeeze your PC muscles during each commercial. Contract the muscles and hold them tight for a slow count to five. At first you might not make it to five, but keep trying. As with any muscle, the more you exercise that muscle, the less effort is required to tighten it and the longer you will be able to keep them tight.

In addition to taking advantage of opportunities in your daily life, set aside specific times when you can be alone at home. Lay down and relax. Starting with a warm bath might help. In your mind, find those PC muscles. Then begin tightening and relaxing five times, each time holding the contraction for a slow count of five. Your goal over a period of time is to increase the number of contractions and the length of time held (although there is a limit to which the PC muscles can be tightened before they automatically begin to relax). Work at it, each time striving to improve your count. If the muscles feel tired, stop and relax for a few seconds and then start in again.

While on your back, also try to do a series of quick Kegels, tightening and relaxing the PC muscles as rapidly as possible, initially five times. Relax for a minute and then do another series of these quick rapid contractions. Work to increase the number of contractions in each series, and work to increase the number of series. You might think of this as "fluttering" your PC muscles. Rest when you need to, but take seriously the challenge of gaining better control over the muscles surrounding the vaginal opening.

It is important to exercise often and it is helpful to add a variety of physical positions. It has also been suggested that it would be helpful to pull in the entire pelvic floor, imagining that you are able to draw water up into your vagina. Then bear down as though you are pushing this imaginary water out. Do that five times to start, and more often as you tone the muscles and increasingly gain strength.

Initially you might want to do the exercises clothed (certainly those series performed on your way to work). At home, however, when you will be comfortable and will have the time, it might be helpful to begin doing the exercises nude.

Combine your "Kegeling" with other activities designed to increase body awareness and sexual sensitivity. You might find that doing your Kegels while masturbating increases the level of your arousal and might even help trigger an orgasm. In fact, there have been a few reports of a small number of woman who have been able to reach orgasm with the vaginal squeeze alone. My advice is not to count on this. Combine the Kegeling with clitoral stimulation and or dildo play.

Kegeling with a Partner

With a partner present and with sufficient arousal and lubrication, have your partner insert two fingers into your vagina. Once inside, your partner should open the fingers up like scissors, and you try to close them with your vaginal sphincter muscles. Repeat this five times on each occasion that you do it. If you are uncomfortable with two fingers, have your partner put in just one and then curl this finger upward.

You try to straighten it out! Invite your man's participation and make it a fun game.

You might also want to use the PC muscles that surround the opening of your vaginal during intercourse, once you are relaxed enough to allow penetration. Grip and relax, grip and relax five times, saying nothing to see if your partner will acknowledge feeling you tighten around him. You could think of it as a flirtatious "vaginal wink." Find joy in learning about your pubococcygeus muscles and share!!

UNDERSTANDING SEX THERAPY

When talking professionally to groups or personally to friends, the question is often asked, "Just what is sex therapy?" and "Exactly what is it you do?" Since these questions occur so often, it was decided to clarify what goes on behind the closed office doors of these specialists.

What Sex Therapy is Not

First, however, it should be clarified what sex therapy is not. Sex therapy is NOT a touching therapy! Like many other non-medical therapies, sex therapy is a talking therapy rather than a touching therapy. At no time can a sex therapist (unless he or she is a physician) request that a person disrobe for a physical examination. Also, clients are never expected to have sex in front of their sex therapist (or counselor) or anywhere while in the office. A sex therapist or counselor is NOT a Sex Surrogate! Sexual techniques are NEVER personally demonstrated or are clients ever touched sexually in any way.

Sex therapy is not a speciality for therapists who are shy when it involves talking about sexual matters. The major difference between sex therapy and other talking therapies is that the talk must go into explicit sexual detail. Specific questions must be asked because it is impossible to help find a solution to sexual concerns without first finding out what is happening sexually in the present, and what occurred sexually in the past. In sex therapy, we realize that it is often easier for clients *to do sex* than *to talk* about it. Therefore, a sex therapist must go to great lengths in trying to put people at ease with talking about sexual issues in general, but also on a very intimate and personal level.

Finally, sex therapy is usually not an individual therapy because most sexual problems do not occur in a vacuum, unless the person is alone. In other words, if a person has a partner, most sexual problems are either created by a person's relationship or have an impact on it. Therefore, the treatment of sexual concerns is most often within the context of a person's relationship. This means that sex therapy is primarily a couples therapy (rather than an individual therapy) and the relationship is the primary focus of treatment. Of course, partners are also treated individually, as needed, and individuals without partners are also counseled for sexual concerns.

It should be pointed out that sex therapy is not the be all and end all when it comes to resolving sexual issues. Sex therapist work closely with urologist, gynecologists and other medical specialists. Sex therapists also, when appropriate, will make referrals to clinicians specializing in issues of sexual abuse, body image concerns, sexual addiction, etc. A sex therapist will also make referrals for sexually unrelated emotional or behavioral concerns.

What Sex Therapy is

Now to answer the first commonly asked question, "What is sex therapy?" By definition, sex therapy is a professional and ethical treatment approach to problems of sexual function and expression. It reflects the recognition that sexuality is a legitimate concern to professionals and that it is the right of individuals to seek expert assistance for their sexual issues and difficulties. Sex therapy focuses on the use of special clinical skills and theoretical knowledge (by the therapist or counselor) to help people attain better sexual expression and achieve more satisfying and fulfilling intimate relationships. It is non-judgmental about the safe behavior of consenting adults, regardless of orientation or marital status.

What clinical skills and body of knowledge does a sex therapist or sex counselor need? First, a sex therapist or counselor must be a licensed psychologist, psychiatrist, professional counselor, clinical social worker or psychiatric nurse. In other words, he or she must be trained and experienced in one of the basic mental health fields, and thereby have extensive knowledge of basic psychotherapy or counseling. Ideally, the sex therapist or counselor should also have additional training in working with couples in marital or relationship counseling because, as mentioned earlier, sexuality is typically a relationship issue. Beyond the basic skills of a mental health practitioner, a sex therapist or counselor needs to have extensive knowledge of the physiological and psychological bases of the sexual response and extensive post-graduate training in sexual function and dysfunction. This training takes years.

It is also necessary for the therapist to be comfort with sexuality, in general and personally, and have an awareness of his or her personal sexual attitudes and biases. A sex therapist or counselor needs to be as free as possible of sexual biases (and other biases) that may adversely affect the objectivity of the therapy. Finally, the sex therapist or counselor must always adhere to a strict professional code of ethics. Not having sex with clients (as previously mentioned) and keeping strict confidentiality are just two of the many ethical codes that guide the profession.

What Occurs in Sex Therapy?

The question, "What is it you do?" will now be explained. The first thing is the assessment and diagnose of the presenting concerns. This includes being able to determine underlying concerns and hidden agendas. Although typically seeing a couple together, there is the option of evaluating each individually. A lot of questions will be asked, but the therapist will also do a great deal of listening. In the process of the evaluation, the therapist must distinguish the difference between biogenic (physical) and psychogenic (psychological) problems and understand how different physical and psychological variables interact. For example, a therapist would not want to spend hours talking to a woman who has sexual pain without being able to first rule out a physical cause such as vaginal dryness, previous vaginal surgery or a size discrepancy. There is also the need to determine if sexual problems are trauma-based, as from sexual abuse (past or present).

Besides questioning and listening, the sex therapist will eventually do a lot of talking. Sex therapy, as it runs its course, becomes a very didactic, directive therapy. That is, it becomes a teaching process using what is known as cognitive/behavioral techniques.

Sex therapists won't usually sit quietly and nod their heads! Since many sexual concerns and problems grow out of sexual ignorance and faulty learning, a lot of preliminary time is spent providing accurate information and correcting faulty assumptions. Specifically, there might be the need to correct sexual myths and gender illusions. Also, a lot of educating about bodies takes place, especially about how bodies function sexually. Any issues of guilt need to be resolved, but within the context of the client's moral belief system.

Often, it is necessary to teach and polish communication skills because to have good sex, effectively communicate is required. Helping with conflict resolution might be involved as the total relationship is addressed. If non-sexual issues exist, the therapist might need to work on relationship issues before starting sex therapy. However, relationship issues and sexual issues can usually be addressed concurrently.

Performance Anxiety

Since anxiety is a common result of sexual difficulties, therapy is often directed toward relieving the fear of failure or apprehension about pain. Following the initial assessment and the establishment of good rapport, specific recommendations are made that become "homework" or "home play." The therapeutic assignment of the Sensate Focus steps is addressed elsewhere in this book.

A therapist will often recommend relevant literature (bibliotherapy) as an adjunct to the therapy. Today there are also a number of educational DVDs that address sexual concerns and promote sensual and sexual intimacy. These educational (and often explicit) programs will be recommended if deemed appropriate.

Sexual Concerns

What kind of sexual concerns do Sex Therapists treat? People seek help for sexual inhibitions, often not encountered until the individual enters a relationship and fails to meet the expectations of a partner.

Other clients present concerns relating to sexual "desire." Most commonly, this relates to desire being too low or to desire that is not in sync with one's partner. This might be a chronic (long-term) concern or could be of more recent onset. There are questions about relationship issues, medications, etc.

Help is also sought for problems of "arousal" (becoming or staying turned on.) Such problems might be expressed as a lack of vaginal lubrication or a man's problem with getting or keeping an erection. There are also concerns with orgasm. Males often express a concern with ejaculating too quickly, although for some it is a problem of delayed ejaculation. Some women have the problems of not reaching orgasm with a partner and at times even when alone. Fortunately, this is less common among women in today's world, given the freer discussion of female sexual anatomy, the availability of vibrators and a growing general awareness of the need for clitoral stimulation.

Sometimes the issue is painful intercourse, due a size discrepancy or the woman cannot have intercourse at all because of involuntary spasms of the vaginal muscles (Vaginismus).

People also bring in concerns of sexual identity and sexual orientation, or for sexual difficulties relating to physical disabilities or illness. Sometimes, people want to simply improve their relationship. The list goes on and on.

Summarizing

The point is, people have the opportunity to take what they have learned in sex therapy and use it as a lifelong investment to build a more satisfying and fulfilling life for themselves and for their mates. To sum up the answer to the question about what a sex therapist does as opposed to a medical doctor who adds years to one's life, the sex therapist works to add life to one's years!

SEXUAL FANTASIES

Have you ever given much thought to the differences between the sexual fantasies typically conjured up by men and by women? Men, it seems, tend to have more sexual fantasies than women and these are more likely to be paired with masturbation. Men, by nature being visual creatures, are likely to create graphic images of women's sexual bodies and imagine watching them, seducing them or, quite often, being seduced by them. For a male, the storyline of a fantasy is usually quite genital and accompanied with explicit visual images.

Women, in general, fantasize less than their male counterparts. Those women who do fantasize are typically less visual in their sexual fantasies, are usually less focused on genitals and are more likely to construct a story with the emotional feelings of a romantic encounter. Women also tend to involve more olfactory and auditory memories – memories of smells and sounds. To be sure, however, there are women who masturbate to their fantasies, be they romantic or erotic.

Sexual fantasies can serve many purposes. They can stir sexual desire, boast and maintain sexual arousal, enhance the sexual experience, trigger an orgasm and preserve a memory.

Lighting the Fire

The desire to be sexual is not something controlled by a switch and easily turned on following the eleven o'clock news. Many people, particularly as they age or as a relationship matures, find that the easy turn ons occur less frequently, particularly late at night. On those occasions when time is limited, fantasies can serve to focus attention on the anticipated erotic event and help induce the desire for sexual intimacy. More than one person has told me, "I'm not able to get excited on a moment's notice. I need time to psych myself up."

To induce desire, you can think ahead about what you would like to experience and what you and your partner will give and receive. Imagine the sexual encounter is your very first, but without those initial anxieties, and let it be, in your mind, a new and exciting adventure. Recall the good sexual feelings you have experienced and mentally reminisce about those most memorable past encounters. Conjure up the memory of a partner's warmth, softness (or hardness) and gentle touch. See your partner's face in your mind's eye and recall that person's sounds of pleasure and the aroma of their excitement. Include only the graphic images you are comfortable with.

Desire can be induced mutually throughout the day, with, for example, a phone call to say, "I've been thinking of your wonderful body." The mid-day message, "You won't believe what I want to do to you tonight," might stir the erotic imagination of both partners, causing each to spend the day thinking of the possibilities in store for that night. Emailing and text messaging offer additional modern day avenues for communicating sexy thoughts and desires.

For those without a partner, fantasies during the day can become the prelude for an episode of self-loving that evening. Self-stimulation, the normal, natural way of experiencing solitary pleasure, is a healthy outlet for many who are alone. Fantasy during the day can certainly prepare you for the quiet celebration of your own sexual response.

Staying on Track

Most of us have had the experience of beginning a sexual encounter, only to find our minds wandering off to the worries of the day or the pressing issues of tomorrow. Erotic fantasy can maintain arousal by pushing away the intrusive nonsexual thoughts. When distractions hit, we need only focus on a pleasant sexual memory or project an exciting visual image on our mental movie screen.

Fantasies can be of our current sexual partner, but often they will revolve around persons from the past, coworkers, movie stars, or attractive strangers. Bringing others into fantasies is normal and is justified if it serves the current relationship by eliminating distractions that would otherwise dampen or destroy the passion.

Obviously, if someone feels guilty about including others in his or her fantasy script, they should be left out. Some people like a cast of hundreds, while others want to focus exclusively on their current partner.

Kinky Content

Many people worry about their fantasies being too far out, but such fantasies are really quite common. Unusual fantasies can help heighten and maintain arousal and are harmless if there is no compulsion to actually experience an act that would be emotionally or physically harmful to oneself or to others. Whereas honesty is usually the best policy, discretion must be used in the sharing of some kinky fantasies or fantasies involving other people. It is rare that a couple can share such deep, dark, private thoughts without, at best, a little discomfort. Too often the reaction upon hearing a partner's most far out fantasy is one of jealousy or distrust, if not anger and disgust.

One woman playfully imagined that her partner's average size penis was enormous, and reported how she would visualize engulfing this gigantic imaginary erection into her body, which in reality would have been quite painful. In her mind she would privately marveled at her vagina's ability to swallow up this massive imaginary tool. She quickly acknowledged, however, that she had no desire to experience anything that large in real life, but she did enjoy embellishing her fantasy with the thoughts of dressing this impressive male member in doll's clothing and taking it for walks in the park. During her sexual encounters, this fantasy helped rivet her attention on the pleasure she was feeling from the very adequate, reasonably-sized penis of her partner.

One night, this woman decided that it would be fun to share her giant penis fantasy with her partner. To her utter surprise, the man was devastated upon hearing her playful musings! He began worrying that she had been with men who had larger penises than his, fearing that these well endowed men must have pleased her more than he could ever hope to do. He erroneously assumed that she could not enjoy his average size penis, and began to feel totally inadequate as her lover. Fearing he could not satisfy this woman, he backed off sexually. When he did try, he felt self-conscious and, as a result, often failed to become erect. This, of course, led to more avoidance and self-degradation.

In couples therapy this man was able to work on understanding that his partner's fantasy had nothing to do with his genital size or sexual performance, but made their shared intimacy more exciting for her. In our last therapy session he began laughing and, when this reaction was questioned, shared his own "pet" fantasy. He had for many years fantasized he was making love to a virgin and that her vagina was the town's tightest. Both agreed that they loved each other, loved the sexuality they shared and would never again ask about the private fantasies each used to dispel the occasional intruding distractions. They also learned that in reality, tight vaginas and large penises are immaterial when a relationship is based on love and mutual respect.

The consequences of disclosure were more serious for another couple. The man fantasized about having sex with his wife's younger married sister. While he found the sister attractive, he had no illusions about her strong commitment to her husband and would never, in reality, make a pass at her. When he shared his fantasy, however, his wife expressed anger and disbelief. She became extremely uncomfortable whenever her sister was around her husband and believed that she had to watch them both closely for any signs of subtle flirtation. Angry that she now felt distrusting, not only of her husband, but of her sister as well, she chose to end her marriage with the man rather than further damage her relationship with her sister. The fantasy proved to be too close, too personal, and too threatening.

Many shared fantasies, however, enhance desire and maintain arousal. One night a man entered a singles bar, propped himself up on a bar stool and slowly rotated, carefully surveying the women around him. Apparently no one caught his eye, so he turned his back on the scene and sipped quietly on his drink. About fifteen minutes later, a woman walked in. As her eyes adjusted to the darkened room, she also scrutinized the crowd. She wandered around a bit, being careful not to make eye contact with any of the men scattered around the room. After a few minutes of aimless wandering, she moved up beside the man who was seemingly intent on nursing his drink. Sliding between him and the person sitting next to him, she leaned toward the bar to catch the bartender's attention. As she did, the man felt her breast brush lightly across his arm, but he did not look her way.

After being served, the woman stepped back, drink in hand, and stood behind the man. Aware of her presence, the man turned and looked into her eyes. His unoriginal inquiry, "Do you come here very often?" was met with an abrupt, "No!" As he turned toward her, his leg came to rest against her thigh. She made no attempt to avoid the contact, but waited for him to continue his attempt to initiate conversation. Awkwardly he asked, "What do you do for fun?" Both grinned at her response, "I pick up strange men in singles bars." At this point the drink he had been nursing so patiently was gulped down in record time and he asked her to dance. She played at being reluctant, but allowed him to convince her. On the dance floor, they danced as though each was covered by porcupine quills and a large man on a Harley-Davidson could have driven between them. As they continued to dance, however, they moved closer until, from a distance, it looked as though their bodies had blended into one.

As they left together he asked, "Shall we take your car or mine?" Again giggling, they took his car to the nearest motel, where he produced a bottle of wine from an ice bucket on the back seat. Ralph and Mary, who had been married for three years, were acting out their shared fantasy. Once in the room, Mary enticed Ralph into seducing her slowly, pretending uncertainty. "I really don't know if I should!" she said coyly as he pretended clumsiness, fumbling to unbutton her blouse and acting bewildered by the complexities of executing the one-handed unsnapping of a push-up bra. During their lovemaking, Mary intentionally cried out, "Oh Bill, you make me feel so good," and that morning, Ralph pretended to have completely forgotten her name. It was a night not soon forgotten, providing the erotic content for many fantasies that followed.

Novelty can get lost in long-term relationships. When a couple becomes comfortable and familiar with each other sexually, they often forget to be romantic. The entire sexual scenario might become routine, taking place at the same time of the day, in the same location, and all too often in a hurry to completion. While it might be impractical for most of us to make love on a beach, in fantasy we can imagine the sound of the ocean, the warmth of the sand beneath our body and the excitement of making love under the stars. Perhaps yours will be a fantasy of making love in the woods, or in an old barn, or in the backseat of the car you had as a teenager.

Some fantasies can be acted out, e.g., a pick up in a grocery store. But most fantasies are just private thoughts that need not have a complex storyline, or a cast of hundreds. Working too hard at building a sexual fantasy can become a distraction, defeating one of its purposes. The best fantasies are often quite simple and tied in with pleasant memories. Often it is visual, creating a mental image of a part of the partner's body that is pleasing to look at, but impossible to see in the dark or in a particular position. At times words can be added to the fantasy while forming the mental image "I love your fantastic buns."

Orgasmic Trigger

Special fantasies can be saved for those times when an orgasm is a bit elusive. These favorites can often add the final bit of excitement needed to trigger a powerful climax. Search your inventory of fantasies. Is there one that is particularly powerful? A favorite that is best saved for the climax? If you discover that you have a springboard fantasy, use it sparingly so as not to wear it out. When you are close to orgasm and hovering on the brink, call up that trigger.

These powerful hot fantasies have been called pet fantasies or trigger fantasies. There are best kept secret and called up only when desperately needed.

The Post-Orgasmic Afterglow

It is nice, in the afterglow of a loving and lustful encounter, to snuggle together and reminisce. Images of the encounter can then be stored for later retrieval to induce desire, maintain arousal, or even trigger an orgasm. Fantasies serve many functions from getting started to getting finished. Remember, sexual fantasies before, during and after a sexual encounter are normal, natural and often helpful in changing a routine experience into a new and exciting event.

THE CALIFORNIA STORY

Illustrating the Concept of Failsafe Sexuality

There was once was a young couple living in New York who, upon meeting, discovered they both loved to travel. Very early in their relationship they began taking trips together and, even without preplanning, they inevitably would wind up in California. They both fell in love with California and together they explored this marvelous place with mutual enthusiasm. Being young, energetic and carefree, they took frequent trips and were never disappointed with the beauty they found and shared at the end of their destination, even though it remained the same.

At some point in their time together, as with most couples in a long-term committed relationship, the frequency of their trips to California decreased. However, they still reveled in the pleasure they found at the end of their cross-county trip to the West Coast. Children had come along, demanding more and more time and energy. Illness at times necessitated the delay of a planned trip, and the stress of work often rendered one or both too tired to even think of packing. But this couple still, whenever possible, made the now less frequent trip to California, and they still loved the beauty of the seacoast.

One night the couple started out, but for the first time in their lives together they ran out of gas along the way. The husband assumed full responsibility, and blamed himself for not having filled the gas tank. He was angry with himself and worried that his car had become too old to make it all the way. He felt he had disappointed his wife and was embarrassed by his sense of failure.

It was obvious they would not complete their trip. "We'll not make it to California," he said, "so we might just as well give up and go home."

"No," said his wife. "We have come this far, so let's get out and explore." Reluctantly her husband agreed, being sure that this place could never be as interesting as California. Together, however, they began to explore and quickly discovered they had run out of gas in Colorado Springs. As they wandered around the area they began to discover many exciting places and, indeed, as they prepared to leave they agreed to begin planning on occasional trips to return to the beauty of these mountains. They had found so much there that they had missed as they dashed through on their rush to California and so they now wanted to come back and, at their leisure, learn about fun things that had been previously ignored.

One night they started out and, for the first time in their lives, they missed a turn. They had driven that highway to California so many times that they often joked they could start the car, head it in the right direction, close their eyes and trust that when they opened them again they would be at their West Coast destination. Now, however, they had gotten off the usual path and seemed hopelessly lost. The wife blamed herself. "If only I had not been distracted," she lamented, "I have failed as our navigator. I should have kept us on track - it was my duty." Disgusted with herself and fearing her husband was disappointed, she suggested they give up and go home.

"No," said her husband, "Let's get out of the car and explore." When they got out, they soon discovered they had somehow ended up in New Orleans. Together, hand in hand, they explored this new Cajun territory, and loved it! They realized now that they had been so focused in the past on getting to California that they had missed the opportunity to explore and experience new and different places. As they got back into their car after their delightful and novel visit, the wife marked the New Orleans exit on their map. They would certainly enjoy coming back to re-experience what they had discovered and to search out even more excitement in this new found city, as well as some stops along the way.

One night they started out and once more ran out of gas. Both looked out of the car windows and realized they were not in Colorado and they were not in Cajun country. The husband spotted a road sign and made out the name of the city - Columbus. In unison, both said, "Let's go home!" However, they remembered the joy they had together in discovering Colorado Springs and in New Orleans and both exclaimed, "Heck, let's get out and explore!" Together they explored and, to their surprise, they had a marvelous time in Ohio's capital city. Columbus joined Colorado Springs and New Orleans on the list of fun places to visit.

This couple continued to take a lot of trips as they aged and the years wore on, and they still could occasionally made it all the way to California. However, their list of other fun places had grown. Salt Lake City, Tulsa, St. Louis, Dallas and many other exciting cites and towns were added, each with its own unique beauty and excitement.

Whenever this couple returned home from a journey, their friends would always ask the very same question, "How was your trip?"

The couple always had the very same answer. "It was fantastic, because we love **traveling** together!" Some of their friends did not understand, as they had never learned to travel. Years ago these friends had run out of gas or gotten off track and could no longer make it all the way to California. They gave up and never again embarked on another trip together!

Moral of the Story

Always remember, California is a wonderful place to visit and should be visited frequently if you can still make the trip. But when you start running out of gas, don't quit your journey and go home. Explore and experience wherever you end up! When you travel together and are enjoying the scenery and the places where you stop to rest, you might still on occasion get back on the road and make it to California. But if you don't, it really doesn't matter! Over a lifetime, you will discover that the **process of traveling** is every bit as much fun as hurrying to reach the destination. Although we will all reach an age where California seems a long way off, **we are never too old to travel!!**

Treating Vaginismus DVD

The DVD opens as a woman tells her partner about the gynecology appointment she had earlier in the day. She explains that the gynecologist diagnosed her condition as "vaginismus" and has referred them as a couple for sex therapy. The film proceeds in the therapist's office with an anatomical explanation of vaginismus. Subsequent sessions introduce the use of dilators in this type of therapy and explains how the woman is to use them in the privacy of her home. Scenes shift between the private sexual sessions at home and the therapist's office. The therapist reviews their progress and provides them with guidelines for additional home sessions. The DVD's conclusion shows the couple successfully engaged in intercourse.

This 30 minute DVD describes in detail the traditional behavioral approach to treating Vaginismus. The presentation is realistic and is explicit. Not all qualified sex therapists will use exactly the same steps, but this DVD gives a woman an understanding of a program that has been used successfully for over thirty years.

Sexual Pain Questionnaire

This is a fourteen-page questionnaire exploring multiple facets of a woman's life for the purpose of pinpointing the cause or causes of sexual pain. The questionnaire was developed by Dr. Robert Birch for use in his clinical practice as is useful as a tool for a woman to consider her situation. It is also help for her to better describe the discomfort she is feeling. It is recommended that the woman take the completed form to her gynecologist or sex therapist, as the responses will aid in the clinical diagnosis of the sexual pain.

The questionnaire is available as a PDF attachment to an email. It can be downloaded with Adobe Acrobat Reader, printed out and completed.

Dildos

On the www.oralcaress.com site you will find a variety of dildos, handpicked for their low price and for their length and circumference.

Vibrating Dildo

Another option for gaining comfort with vaginal penetration is the use of a vibrating dildo. Used alternately on the clitoris and vaginally, this allow for maintaining arousal during the relaxation and exploration session. Most are only 1 inch in diameter to allow easy entry.

Astroglide

Astroglide is one of the most popular sexual lubricants on the market, and is considered by many to be second only to nature. With difficult penetration, related to partner size, vaginal dryness or both, ample lubrication is recommended. Astroglide mixes readily with a woman's natural lubrication, will not harm latex, and washes off easily.

A Guide to Female Orgasm During Intercourse

Getting comfortable and now wondering about orgasms during intercourse? Then consider the illustrated articles available as PDF files on a data CD.

Find it among the many exciting and educational resources at http://www.oralcaress.com. Dr. Birch, author of this book and host of the website, is available to answer questions. His email address is birchbarks@aol.com.

FINDING A SEXUALITY THERAPIST

If you or your partner are thinking that it might help to talk with a therapist, or if your relationship is in trouble because of your orgasmic or other sexual concerns, do not hesitate to consult a qualified sexuality therapist or counselor. If there are no other relationship issues, a well trained and experienced sex therapist can assist you in a relatively brief period of time. To locate a qualified professional in your geographic area, visit the website or write to one or both of the following national certificating associations:

American Association of Sex Educators, Counselors and Therapists (AASECT)
  P.O. Box 1960
  Ashland, VA 23005-1960
  Phone: 804.752.0026, Fax: 804.752.0056,
    e-Mail: aasect@aasect.org
    Web site: **http://www.aasect.org**

American Academy of Clinical Sexologists (AACS)
  1929 18th Street, N.W., Suite 1166
  Washington DC 20009
  Phone: 202.462.2122

The American Board of Sexology
  3203 Lawton Road, Suite 170
  Orlando FL 32803
  Phone: 407.574.5708, FAX 407.574.8943

To find additional professional assistance in your geographical area, check the roster of qualified sexuality therapists and counselors through the listing of the Institute for Marital and Sex Therapy. **http://www.sexualtherapy.com**

_____Also, check out the listing of qualified professionals on the website of the Society for Sex Therapy and Research, on the web at. **http://www.sstarnet.org/directory.cfm**

ABOUT THE AUTHOR

__Robert W. Birch, Ph.D.__, certified sexologist and adult sexuality educator, is now retired, but had maintained an independent psychological practice, specializing in marital, family and sex therapy for well over 35 years. Dr. Birch received his Bachelors Degree from Muskingum College in 1960, his Masters Degree from the Ohio University in 1962, and his Ph.D. from the University of Wisconsin in 1967.

He has been a sex therapy consultant to the Medical Center at Wright-Patterson Air Force Base, has been an adjunct faculty member in the Ohio University Psychology Department and in the Ohio State University Family Therapy program. Dr. Birch has served on the national board of directors of the American Association for Marriage and Family Therapy (AAMFT), the American Association of Sex Educators, Counselors and Therapists (AASECT), and the Board of Examiners of the American Board of Family Psychology.

Dr. Birch was the first Certified Sex Therapist in the State of Ohio. Before his retirement, he had been certified by AASECT as a Sex Therapist, Sex Educator and Supervisor and was a Clinical Member, Fellow and Approved Supervisor of AAMFT. He was certified as a Family Therapist by the National Alliance of Certified Family Therapists, and was certified as a Sex Therapist and Supervisor by the American Board of Sexology. He was a Founding Fellow of the American Academy of Clinical Sexologists, a Fellow of the American Academy of Family Psychology, and a Diplomate of the American Board of Family Psychology. He holds a lifetime certification as Sexologist by the American College of Sexologists.

Dr. Birch has presented over 350 guest lectures and lead over 100 professional workshops and seminars. He has served as the Audio-Visual Review Editor of the *Journal of Sex Education and Therapy* as well as being on the Editorial Board of that journal and of the *Journal of Family Therapy*. He is the coauthor of a chapter on Female Sexual Concerns in a book titled *Twenty Common Health Concerns of Women*. He had been a regular guest on radio and TV and continues to be interviewed for national magazines.

Dr. Birch believes that our sexuality is a gift to be enjoyed by consenting adults in loving ways, but never taken too seriously, lest we forget that sex is supposed to be fun. In his retirement he has moved to rural Ohio where he continues to write (with wisdom and wit) in the company of his wife Susan, four dogs, two cats and a very spoiled cockatiel named George.

OTHER SEXUALITY
SELF-HELP BOOKS BY THE AUTHOR

ORAL CARESS: The Loving Guide to Exciting a Woman
1-57074-307-X, 1996

CUNNILINGUS: Warm Her Heart and Tickle Her Pink
1-57074-500-5, 2006

A SEX THERAPIST'S MANUAL: Resources for Clinical or
Educational Use 1-57074-320-7, 1996

MALE SEXUAL ENDURANCE: A Man's Book about
Ejaculatory Control 1-57074-349-5, 1997

SENSUAL PATHWAYS TO PLEASURE: A Woman's Journey
to Orgasm, Coauthored by Cynthia Lief Ruberg,
0-55703-823-5, 2006

SEX AND THE AGING MALE: Understanding and Coping
with Change 1-57074-482-3, 2000

A SHORT BOOK ABOUT LASTING LONGER: Step by Step
Basics for the Management of Premature Ejaculation
1-57074-486-6, 2001

WHAT I KNOW ABOUT SEX: Problems and Pleasures
1-45152-862-0, 2010

These books are available from the author's website at
www.oralcaress.com or on Amazon.com.